SEX, LOVE AND HEDONISM

Amy Mandeville

Additional material by Rachael Osborne

Summersdale Publishers Ltd
46 West Street
Chichester
West Sussex
PO19 1RP

www.summersdale.com

Printed and bound in Great Britain.

ISBN 184024 119 5

CONTENTS

DEFINITIONS

sex

Etymology: Middle English, from Latin *sexus*

1: the sum of the characteristics that distinguish an animal or plant as male or female

2 a: sexually motivated phenomena or behaviour

b: sexual intercourse

3: genitalia

love

Etymology: Middle English, from Old English *lufu* love; akin to Old High German *luba* love; Old English *leof* dear; Latin *lubet* it pleases

1 (a): strong affection for another arising out of kinship or personal ties (b): attraction based on sexual desire: affection and tenderness felt by lovers (c): affection based on admiration, benevolence, or common interests

2: warm attachment, enthusiasm, or devotion

3: a beloved person; often used as a term of endearment

4: an amorous episode: love affair

5: the sexual embrace: copulation

hedonism

Etymology: Greek, from *hçdonç* pleasure

1: the doctrine that pleasure or happiness is the sole or chief good in life

2: a way of life based on or suggesting the principles of hedonism

Welcome to a little book devoted entirely to the realms of passion, love and the erotic. Whether devoured from cover to cover in one sitting, or dipped into when the mood takes you, you will find everything essential for the sensual life between these covers.

Sex, love and hedonism are eminently compatible and have always had an intertwined relationship. Complementing each other perfectly, they exemplify the finer things in life and should frequently be indulged in to ensure you get everything out of life that you deserve.

From the myths and legends of the ancients to stories of some of the hedonists of more recent history, and from cooking erotic feasts and giving a great massage to inspiring poetry, your pleasure threshold will be raised and your carnal and romantic wellbeing enriched with these irresistible pages.

. . . THROUGH THE AGES . . .

The Gregarious Greeks

Where better to start than at some of the very first instances of sex, love and hedonism? Passed down by word of mouth through generations of people and over many hundreds of years, Greek mythology has inspired some of the world's most romantic stories. Often identified with their Roman equivalents, the Greek gods were well-known for their excesses – whether of the lustful or gluttonous kind.

Zeus was the greatest of the Greek gods and, being a god of fertility, the most amorous. He was king of the heavens and earth, rewarding good and punishing evil. Here are some of his conquests . . .

Zeus and . . .

. . . Semele

Zeus set his sights on the Theban princess Semele. He made himself invisible and, seducing her through touch alone, slept with her. Semele became pregnant with a son, Dionysus.

Hera, Zeus' jealous wife, on learning of his infidelity and well aware of the shock it would cause demanded that Zeus show himself to Semele. He appeared before her as a lightning bolt and the six-months pregnant Semele died of fright. Zeus, heartbroken, saved the baby. Dionysus was sewn into Zeus' thigh until he was ready to be born and Dionysus became known as 'twice-born.'

. . . Leto

Another story involves Zeus' dalliance with the beautiful Leto. On the lovers coupling, Zeus turned them both into quails.

In retaliation for her husband's straying, Hera sent the serpent Python to pursue Leto who was pregnant with twins.

Zeus saved her by sending the North Wind to

carry her over the sea to the Greek island of Delos. Here, Leto bore Artemis, who helped her travel further from Hera's wrath, and Apollo was born nine days later.

. . . Io

According to lore, Zeus fell in love with Io. In order to seduce her whilst hidden from Hera, Zeus covered the world in a blanket of clouds.

But Hera became suspicious, and appeared through the clouds, whereupon Zeus swiftly turned Io into a white cow. Unconvinced by his tricks, Hera sent the cow to be watched over by Argus Panoptes, a creature with a hundred eyes, to ensure that Io would remain in cow form forever.

Zeus then employed the greatest musician, Hermes, to sing Argus Panoptes to sleep, so he could be killed. Io thus escaped and after many adventures, was finally turned back into a woman by Zeus.

Theseus and Ariadne

Tyrannical King Minos of Crete decreed to Aegeus, the king of Athens, that he would wage war unless seven men and seven women were sent to combat the Minotaur every year.

The Minotaur was a fearsome creature, half man and half bull, who lived in a pitch-black labyrinth under the castle.

Theseus, the son of the king of Athens, volunteered to go and kill the Minotaur. Once in Crete he met and fell in love with Ariadne, the king's daughter, who gave him a ball of twine to lead him out of the maze and a magic sword with which to kill the Minotaur. After he had defeated the beast, he took Ariadne with him on the ship back to Athens. On the journey he dreamed that she was destined to become the wife of a god and so, believing the oracle, he left her on the island of Naxos while she was asleep.

In his sorrow at what he had done, Theseus forgot his promise to his father; that he would hoist a white sail if his endeavours were successful. Coming into harbour with the original black sails, Aegeus threw himself to his death in the sea, believing that his son had perished.

Pygmalion and Galatea

Pygmalion, king of Cyprus, was a gifted sculptor who spurned all women for Galatea, a beautiful statue he had sculpted and robed in fine clothes and jewels. He longed for her to be real. The dejected artist appealed to the goddess Aphrodite who, much to his surprise, breathed life into his Galatea, ensuring the couple an enduring happiness.

Helen and Paris

The most handsome of mortal men, Paris was chosen

to judge a beauty contest between the three loveliest goddesses. Hera offered him wealth if she was picked, Athena, patron goddess of Athens, promised him success in war, and Aphrodite pledged to grant him the most beautiful of mortal women for his wife.

Paris chose Aphrodite, who then assisted him in his abduction of Helen (the face that launched a thousand ships) who was already married to the Greek king Menelaus. The ensuing war that occurred between the Greeks and Trojans because of both men's love for Helen lasted ten years and is the most famous in classical mythology.

Eros and Psyche

Aphrodite, the mother of Eros, was so jealous of the mortal Psyche's beauty that she ordered her son to pierce the girl's heart with an arrow and cause her to fall in love with a man who would give her a lifetime of grief.

Eros went to do his mother's bidding, but was astonished by Psyche's beauty and dropped the arrow which pierced his foot, causing him to fall powerfully in love with the girl.

After wandering in lovesick despair, Eros had

Psyche brought to his home, where she was granted everything but a viewing of his face and form. Too tempted to resist, she finally stole a look at him, and, on being seen by a mortal, Eros was compelled to fly away.

However, Eros saved Psyche once again from his mother's rage and, with his love, made her immortal.

Orpheus and Eurydice

Eurydice, beloved wife of Orpheus, was fatally bitten by a serpent and descended into the Underworld. With the aid of his lute, the mourning Orpheus persuaded Hades, king of the Underworld, to let his wife go.

Hades complied on one condition: that he did not look back at his wife as they ascended into the world again. At the mouth of the Underworld, however, Orpheus gave in to temptation and turned to ensure that his wife really was following him. Instantly, Eurydice was sucked back into the bowels of the earth.

Unable to bear their separation or his mistake, Orpheus pined to death and quickly followed his bride into the Underworld.

Echo and Narcissus

As soon as he was born, Narcissus' mother took him to a prophet who told her that he would live to old age as long as he did not come to know his own image. Terrified, his mother broke every mirror she could to prevent her son from seeing himself.

As he grew up, Narcissus became extremely handsome. He was beloved by all women and became incurably vain.

One day, whilst walking in a woody glade, the nymph Echo spied Narcissus and immediately fell in love with him. However, Echo had to bear a curse, and was only able to repeat what others said. Hearing a rustle in the branches, Narcissus called out, 'What brings you?' 'You!' replied Echo, unable to talk to the object of her love. 'There can be nothing between you and Narcissus!' the young man cried. 'Narcissus!' wept Echo.

Lost in the wood now, Narcissus lay by a pool and caught sight of his own reflection in the water. Enchanted and instantly in love, he looked closer and was amazed to see that the figure in the water leaned towards him. No matter how hard he tried, he couldn't reach his new beloved, and he wasted away by the water, the gods turning him into the fragrant flower that bears his name.

As for Echo, she also suffered unrequited love and now only her voice remains among the rocks.

Aphrodite

Goddess of passion, sex and beauty, born of sea foam and emerging from the shell of a clam, Venus was the most beautiful of all goddesses. Some legends say she came from the foam that gathered around the genitals of Uranus, while others say she was another child of Zeus.

Generally kind and generous to those she favoured, she was vindictive and vicious with those who didn't comply with her will. She was particularly malicious with mortal women rumoured to be as beautiful as her.

Dionysus

Fathered by the wandering Zeus and the mortal Semele, Dionysus had a rich and full demi-godhood during which he invented wine and specialised in driving people insane with pleasure and debauchery, before ascending to Olympus to become one of Zeus' right-hand gods. He was said to suffer greatly in the winter when the vines withered. His mortal followers consumed great quantities of wine and lived for their hedonistic partying.

POETRY

Sexy Stanzas

Passing stranger!
you do not know how longingly I look upon you,
You must be he I was seeking, or she I was seeking,
(it comes to me as if in a dream).
I have somewhere surely lived a life of joy with you,
All is recall'd as we flit by each other,
fluid, affectionate, chaste, matured.
You grew up with me,
were a boy with me or a girl with me,
I ate with you and slept with you –
Your body has become not yours only
nor left my body mine only.

You give me the pleasure of your eyes,
face, flesh, as we pass –
You take of my face, breast, hands in return,
I am not to speak to you
– I am to think of you when I sit alone
or wake at night alone,
I am to wait, I do not doubt I am to meet you again,
I am to see to it that I do not lose you.

Walt Whitman
from *To A Stranger*

Now therefore, while the youthful hue
Sits on thy skin like morning dew,
And while thy willing soul transpires
At every pore with instant fires,
Now let us sport us while we may;
And now, like am'rous birds of prey,
Rather at once our time devour,

Than languish in his slow-chapp'd power.
Let us roll all our strength and all
Our sweetness up into one ball;
And tear our pleasures with rough strife
Thorough the iron gates of life.
Thus, though we cannot make our sun
Stand still, yet we will make him run.

Andrew Marvell
from *To His Coy Mistress*

Away with silks, away with lawn,
I'll have no screens or curtains drawn.
Give me my mistress, as she is,
Dressed in her naked simplicities:
For as my heart, e'en so mine eye,
Is won with flesh, not drapery.

Robert Herrick
from *Clothes Do But Cheat and Cozen Us*

License my roving hands, and let them go
Before, behind, between, above, and below.
O my America, my Newfoundland,
My kingdom, safest when with one man manned,
My mine of precious stones, my empery;
How am I blest in thus discovering thee!
To enter in these bonds, is to be free;
Then, where my hand is set, my soul shall be.
Full nakedness! All joys are due to thee;
As souls unbodied, bodies unclothed must be
To taste whole joys.

John Donne

from *On His Mistress Going to Bed*

Gather ye Rose-buds while ye may,
Old Time is still a-flying:
And this same flower that smiles today,
Tomorrow will be dying.

That Age is best which is the first,
When Youth and Blood are warmer;
But being spent, the worse, and worst
Times still succeed the former.

Then be not coy, but use your time,
And while ye may, go marry;
For having lost but once your prime,
You may forever tarry.

Robert Herrick

from *To The Virgins, to Make Much of Time*

You think it horrible that lust and rage
Should dance attention upon my old age;
They were not such a plague when I was young;
What else have I to spur me into song?

William Butler Yeats
from *The Spur*

Loving Lyrics

I, who have love and no more,
Bring you but love of you, sweet.
He that hath more, let him give;
He that hath wings, let him soar:
Mine is the heart at your feet
Here, that must love you to live.

Algernon Charles Swinburne

from *Obligation*

Then farewell love, and farewell woe,
I will no longer pine;
For I'll believe I have her heart
As much as she hath mine.

Sir John Suckling

from *The Stolen Heart*

Trusty, dusky, vivid, true
With eyes of gold and bramble-dew,
Steel-true and blade-straight,
The great artificer
Made my mate.

Robert Louis Stevenson

from *My Wife*

One hour with thee! When sun is set,
Oh, what can teach me to forget
The thankless labours of the day;
The hopes, the wishes, flung away;
The increasing wants, and lessening gains,
The master's pride, who scorns my pains?
One hour with thee.

Sir Walter Scott

from *An Hour With Thee*

Come to me in the silence of the night;
Come in the speaking silence of a dream;
Come with the soft rounded cheeks and eyes as bright
As sunlight on a stream;
Come back in tears;
Oh memory, hope, love of finished years.

Christina Rossetti

from *Echo*

Oh, no – not ev'n when first we lov'd
Wert thou as dear as now thou art;
Thy beauty then my senses mov'd
But now thy virtues bind my heart.
What was but Passion's sigh before
Has since been turn'd to Reason's vow;
And, though I then might love thee more,
Trust me, I love thee better now.

Thomas Moore

from *Oh, No – Not Ev'n When we First Lov'd*

Drink to me, only, with thine eyes,
And I will pledge with mine;
Or leave a kiss but in the cup
And I'll not look for wine.
The thirst that from the soul doth rise
Doth ask a drink divine;
But might I of Jove's nectar sup
I would not change for thine.

Ben Johnson

from *To Celia*

Thou art my life, my love, my heart,
The very eyes of me;
And hast command of every part,
To live and die for thee.

Robert Herrick

from *To Anthea*

I love my love in the morning,
I love my love at even;
Her smile's soft play is like the ray
That lights the western heaven:
I loved her when the sun was high,
I loved her when he rose;
But best of all when evening's sigh
Was murmuring at its close.

Gerald Griffin

from *I Love My Love in the Morning*

Poems for Pleasure Lovers

Let us have wine and women, mirth and laughter,
Sermons and soda water the day after.

Lord Byron

from *Don Juan*

Wine comes in at the mouth

And love comes in at the eye;

That's all we shall know for truth

Before we grow old and die.

William Butler Yeats

from *A Drinking Song*

If all be true that I do think,
There are five reasons we should drink:
Good wine – a friend – or being dry –
Or lest we should be by and by –
Or any other reason why.

Henry Aldrich

Five Reasons for Drinking

He who does not love wine, women and song
Remains a fool his whole life long.

Johann Heinrich Voss

On with the dance! let joy be unconfined;
No sleep till morn, when Youth and Pleasure meet
To chase the glowing hours with flying feet.

Lord Byron

from *Childe Harold's Pilgrimage*

There was a young fellow named Meek,
Who invented a lingual technique;
It drove women frantic,
And made them romantic,
And wore all the hair off his cheek.

Anonymous

Have ye beheld (with much delight)
A red rose peeping through a white?
Or else a cherry, double graced,
Within a lily centre plac'd?
Or ever marked the pretty beam
A strawberry shows half-drown'd in cream?
Or seen rich rubies blushing through
A pure smooth pearl and orient too?
So like to this, nay all the rest,
Is each neat niplet of her breast.

Robert Herrick

From, *Upon the Nipples of Julia's Breast*

There were once two young people of taste
Who were beautiful down to the waist.
So they limited love
To the regions above,
And thus remained perfectly chaste.

Anonymous

'I DO!'

– Wedding Traditions from Around the World

Weddings. You either love them or dread them. But as you gaze at the bride in envy or pity, have you ever wondered why she must wear 'something old, something new, something borrowed and something blue'? Here are some of the world's more unusual wedding rituals, and their explanations.

African

During the wedding ceremony, the couple's hands are bound at the wrists, literally 'tying the knot'.

In South Africa, the parents of the bride and groom carry a fire from the hearths of their own homes to the couple's home to ensure that the light and warmth continue through the generations.

American Indian

Before the wedding ceremony, the couple must wash their hands to symbolically cleanse themselves of any past lovers they might have had.

Chinese

Wedding invitations and gifts of money to the newlyweds are sent in red envelopes, the traditional colour of wealth and happiness. After the ceremony, fireworks are let off to keep evil spirits away.

Cuban

In Cuba, each man that dances with the bride at the wedding reception has to pin money on to her dress.

Czech

There are two Czech traditions to enhance fertility. The bridesmaids pin rosemary on the wedding guests, and a baby or child is briefly placed on the couple's bed on the wedding night.

Dutch

Lily-of-the-valley is planted in the couple's garden to remind them of their wedding vows as it blooms every year.

English

An English bride must wear 'something old, something new, something borrowed and something blue'. The old and new items represent the transition from being single to the new status of being married. The borrowed item symbolises the participation and approval of the wedding by family and friends. Blue is a symbol of purity, love and fidelity.

Brides toss their bouquets because it is said that the single woman who catches the bouquet is the one who receives the bride's good fortune and will marry next.

It was considered good luck if a chimney sweep kissed a bride on her way to church.

Filipino

In the Philippines, the bride and groom release a pair of doves from an ornate bell made of flowers to symbolise their love.

French

Guests will bang pots and pans and sing loudly outside the couple's room during the wedding night until the groom invites them in for drinks and snacks. This is symbolic of the continuing friendship between the guests and the groom, despite his heart belonging to his wife.

Italian

In Italy, the groom's tie is cut into pieces and sold to the guests at the reception. The money earned is put towards the honeymoon.

Japanese

Ducks or a goose and gander are included in the Japanese wedding procession because they mate for life and are symbols of fidelity.

Jewish

The Jewish wedding ceremony usually takes place under a *huppah*, or wedding canopy. This tradition began in the Middle Ages when a couple would wed outdoors so that the marriage could be blessed with as many children as there are stars in the heavens.

Korean

At a Korean wedding, the groom's father tosses red dates towards the bride, to show his hope for many grandchildren. The bride wears a large red dot on each cheek to ward off evil spirits or demons.

Lithuanian

At a Lithuanian wedding reception, the couple are given the 'elements of life'. These are bread and salt, so they will never go hungry, and wine and honey to ensure that their life together is full of good things.

Mexican

In Mexico, the groom presents thirteen gold coins to his bride as his promise to support her. The *arras*, a small chest of coins symbolising wealth and strength, is blessed during their ceremony.

Moravian

The Moravian Wedding Ritual is a simple but effective romantic gesture. The bride and groom light a large candle together and the flame is passed along to the first guest, who uses the flame to light their own candle. The guest lights their neighbour's candle and so on until everyone is holding a lit candle, showering the party in a warm glow.

Polish

On the way to church, the Polish bride and groom are blocked by children to whom the best man must pay a toll.

Quaker

Quaker tradition does not include clergy, so the wedding certificate is not only signed by the bride and groom, maid of honour and best man, but every single guest signs as witnesses. The wedding certificate is hung in a prominent place in the couple's house, reminding them of the love and support of their family and friends.

The bride presents herself to the groom, rather than being given away by her father, for Quakers believe that she belongs to no one but herself.

Russian

On her wedding day, the bride asks her parents for forgiveness for any offences she may have caused. Her parents present the bride with bread and salt, in the hopes that she will never want for food.

To show their preference of the sex of their first child, the newlyweds tie a doll for a girl or a bear for a boy to the front of their wedding car.

Vietnamese

In Vietnam, the groom leads a procession to the bride's house, picking up family and friends along the way. When they arrive, they give the bride gifts of clothes, jewellery and money. The groom's mother does not join the procession, to show the bride that there is no rivalry between them.

LATE LOVERS

Casanova (1725 – 1798)

The most (in)famous lover in history, by his own count Casanova slept with 10,000 women. The man whose name is now synonymous with 'libertine', Casanova's career spanned from being a violinist in Venice to introducing the lottery in Paris.

On the subject of the lottery, although he used a pig's bladder to protect from pregnancy, he was known to have fathered two daughters: both of whom he had incestuous affairs with.

However, despite his reputation with women, he was also an active homosexual.

His last words were, 'I have lived as a philosopher and die as a Christian.'

Charles Dickens (1812 – 1870)

Although not immediately associated with sex, love or hedonism, Dickens had a fascinating love life. It seems that he had a yen for one particular family of sisters. He married Catherine Hogarth and yet proceeded to fall in love with her seventeen-year-old sister Mary, whom he moved into his household. Distraught when she died in his arms, he eventually separated from his wife and was rumoured to have had an affair with another sister, Georgina.

Charles II (1630 – 1685)

Charles' reign was the era of 'Merrie Olde England'. Extravagant, and a man whose primary indulgence was women, Charles was known to have had at least thirteen mistresses (all of whom, save one, were Catholic). He was said to enjoy, as one wit of the day noted, 'both types of mutton – sheep and loose women'.

Catherine The Great (1729 – 1796)

Catherine became the Empress of Russia through her marriage to Tsar Peter III. Unfortunately for the Tsar, he contracted small pox which left him pockmarked and with very little hair. This, along with the fact that he tried to make his mistress his wife, makes it more understandable that Catherine had twenty-one official lovers and probably many more 'unofficial' ones.

Catherine and her lover Count Gregory Orlov overthrew Peter III and she ruled Russia for thirty-four years, making it her mission to many more schools and hospitals to cover her vast country.

There is speculation that she may secretly have married another lover, Gregory Potemkin, whom she made a Prince of the Empire.

Wallis Simpson (1896 – 1986)

This American divorcée famously tempted a British king from his throne, some said for her bedroom talents. Simpson, who was rumoured to have had a string of lovers before catching the eye of Edward VIII, was said to have learned her skills in the brothels of Shanghai.

She was at other times rumoured to be a man, and to have had a long-standing affair with the homosexual Florida millionaire, Jimmy Donahue, the grandson of F. W. Woolworth. Donahue apparently funded the glamorous lifestyle of the pair. Whatever the truth, Simpson's attentions to the abdicated monarch were enough to keep him by her side for as long as the couple shared time on earth.

John F. Kennedy (1917 – 1963)

Like his father and grandfather before him, John F. Kennedy, the golden boy and slain son of American politics, was renowned for his fondness for women. It was common knowledge among his staff that he would frequently swim naked with two of his secretaries at lunchtime. He also had an affair with a gangster's moll and a possible German spy during the course of his presidency – indiscretions that would have sunk him in today's political climate.

His relationship with Marilyn Monroe as well as other Hollywood starlets is now legendary. He did not, however, keep Monroe to himself – he shared Hollywood's favourite blonde with his brother Robert.

Mae West (1892 – 1980)

The American actress and mistress of the double entendre, West was best known for her portrayals of flamboyant women of lost virtue and few regrets. Censorship had toned down her brazenly sexy film characters in movies such as *Night After Night* (1931) and *I'm No Angel* (1933) and she eventually left the cinema as a creative outlet. Later she worked mainly onstage, notably in her Broadway play, *Catherine Was Great* (1944).

It was during a performance that she coined the phrase, 'Is that a sword in your pocket or are you happy to see me?' Today Mae West is generally known as the woman who brought sexuality out of the bedroom and on to the silver screen.

ROMANTICS REMEMBERED

Elizabeth Barrett Browning and Robert Browning

Elizabeth Barrett, who would in time become a famous romantic poet, spent much of her youth as an invalid in her domineering father's London house. Browning had pledged his love to Barrett before he had even laid eyes on her, having been smitten by her poetry.

After several months of secretive courtship the couple managed to smuggle Barrett out of the house for good. The two lived out their lives together in the warmer climate of Italy and had a child. Elizabeth died in Robert's arms after fifteen years of marriage. Ten years after her death he was heard to say, 'The simple truth is that she was the poet and I the clever person by comparison.'

Romeo and Juliet

Shakespeare's *Romeo and Juliet* is based on a much older tale of uncertain origin and tells the story of youthful and all-encompassing love between a pair of teenagers from opposing families. The couple, knowing their love was prohibited, married secretly. Yet due to a number of misunderstandings, the pair died by their own hands inside Juliet's family tomb. This proved enough of a catalyst to mend the family feud.

Heloïse and Abelard

Abelard, a gifted teacher in medieval Paris, had admired the beautiful and brilliant Heloïse for a long time. Heloïse's uncle was Canon of Notre Dame, and Abelard soon convinced the canon to let him share his home in exchange for instructing the willing Heloïse. Their tentative romance soon blossomed into passion, and it didn't take Uncle Fulbert long to learn of the situation. The pair were parted, but another problem soon arose: Heloïse was pregnant.

The couple fled to the home of Abelard's family, where she gave birth to a son. Upon their return, the pair were married despite the objections of Heloïse, who feared the union would ruin Abelard's career. Her uncle was furious and beat her. For her safety, Abelard sent her to a convent. This proved a terrible mistake. Fulbert, assuming Abelard was trying to unload his new bride, had the groom castrated.

Abelard and Heloïse both took the cloth, but remained in close contact throughout their lives. Upon their deaths they were buried next to each other. Their tomb can be seen at the Père Lachaise, the celebrated burial ground in Paris.

Antony and Cleopatra

Queen of Egypt in the first century BC, Cleopatra seduced the dictator of Rome, Julius Caesar, to consolidate her political power. He erected a golden statue of her in Rome, to prove his love. Caesar was murdered in 44 BC and Cleopatra turned her affections to Mark Antony. Meeting him in Tarsus, she sailed up the Cydnus River resplendent in a beautiful boat, the meeting later immortalised by Shakespeare. Forgetting his wife in Italy, Antony was smitten.

But the Romans turned against Antony and their relationship was doomed. He fell on his sword and Cleopatra, lying on a bed of gold in her royal finery, died from the bite of an asp, the symbol of divine royalty. Whether her first son, whom she called Caesarion, was Caesar's is still unknown.

Victoria and Albert

Prince Albert, husband of Queen Victoria, is widely rumoured to have been so well-endowed that he required a ring set in his penis through which a gold chain could be threaded to keep it in place.

Victoria and Albert were profoundly in love and enjoyed a very happy marriage, producing nine children in their twenty-one years together. When Albert died, Victoria wore mourning clothes for the rest of her life and insisted Albert's clothes be laid out on the bed every morning.

HEDONISTS FROM HISTORY

F. Scott Fitzgerald and Zelda Sayre Fitzgerald

A pair of heroic lovers and hedonists, Fitzgerald said of Zelda, 'I fell in love with a whirlwind.' The pair epitomised the roaring twenties with their free spending, alcoholism, drug addiction, and adultery. They were thrown out of their honeymoon hotel because of their rowdiness. Their parties were legendary, with house rules such as, 'Visitors are requested not to break down the doors in search of liquor, even when authorised to do so by the host and hostess.'

Despite extramarital affairs with several famous contemporaries and numerous prostitutes, Fitzgerald's heart belonged to Zelda, who was diagnosed as a schizophrenic nine years after the marriage. The pair had one daughter, Scotty.

Their gravestone reads, 'So we beat on, boats against the current, borne back ceaselessly into the past.' The line is the last from *The Great Gatsby*.

Lord Byron (1788 – 1824)

One of the great romantic poets, Byron's name has become synonymous with sex, love and hedonism. Born with a club foot, Byron grew to be irresistibly attractive and was a known bisexual who participated in a number of affairs with both men and women. He had relationships with Shelley's sister-in-law and Caroline Lamb who famously called him 'mad, bad and dangerous to know.'

His exploits include drinking red wine out of a human skull and while at Cambridge he kept a bear because dogs were prohibited.

Messalina (22 – 48)

Messalina, the wife of the Roman Emperor Claudius, kept a room at a bordello where she entertained clients and satisfied her sexual appetite and curiosity. Messalina publicly married her lover, Caius Silius, while Claudius was away. Humiliated before his Roman citizens, Claudius had her executed. Her name has become a byword for avarice, lust and cruelty.

Marquis De Sade (1740 – 1814)

The man whose name gave language the word 'sadism' was arrested for the first time for *débauché outrée* just six months after his wedding. He was bisexual and kept a number of mistresses as well as regularly having sex with his manservant, who participated in De Sade's orgies. He frequently hired prostitutes for the purpose of flogging them, and participated in all varieties of sex, allegedly whether the partner was willing or not. De Sade was later imprisoned for inflicting grievous bodily harm by flogging, and again in 1772 for 'unnatural offences'. He spent a total of twenty-seven years in prisons or asylums.

Leopold Von Sacher-Masoch (1836 – 1895)

Sacher-Masoch, the origin of the word 'masochist', was a highly intelligent young man, receiving his law degree aged just nineteen. The Austrian novelist wrote tales of men being flogged, sexually dominated and getting pleasure from the pain they inflicted upon themselves. His most famous book, *Venus in Furs*, procured him notoriety and his eventual place in the English language.

A quiet and amiable man who adored his children, his hedonism only stretched to sex: he never smoked or drank.

Ivan the Terrible (1530 – 1584)

Ivan, Tsar of Russia, kept numerous mistresses and was married seven times, disposing of his wives by forcing them to take the veil (becoming nuns) or having them murdered. He was known to enjoy sexual indulgences of all sorts. He drank to excess and was only ever seen to laugh when watching someone be tortured. He had Prince Shuisky eaten alive by his own dogs, nailed a French envoy's hat to the man's head and killed his own son in a fit of rage.

Tallulah Bankhead (1902 – 1968)

Tallulah Bankhead was romantically linked with many of the luminaries of her time, both male and female. Allegedly, these included John Barrymore Sr., Robert Benchley, Leonard Bernstein, Marlon Brando, Yul Brynner, Winston Churchill, Gary Cooper, Greta Garbo and Billie Holiday. Tallulah's father was the prominent political figure William Brockman Bankhead. Tallulah is frequently quoted as saying, 'My father warned me about men and booze but he never mentioned a word about women and cocaine.' She was famous for her excessive involvement in both, as well as for her habit of drinking two bottles of whisky a day.

Caligula (12 – 41)

Philo catalogued the preferences of the Roman Emperor Caligula as: 'heavy drinking and a taste for delicacies, an insatiable appetite even on a swollen stomach, hot baths at the wrong time, emetics followed immediately by further drinking and the gluttony that goes with it, indecent behaviour with boys and women, and all the vices which destroy the body and soul and the bonds which unite them simultaneously.' Caligula was murdered and buried in a shallow grave having killed most of his family and many of his sexual conquests.

. . . IN PRACTICE . . .

The Science of Love

What is it that makes us fall for a particular person? Why do we always go for certain 'types'? Some believe that we are attracted to people who are like our mothers and fathers, others argue that we fall in love with those who are the *opposite* of our parents. Before dismissing the science as unromantic and placing trust in chance meetings that were 'meant to be', is there more to sexual chemistry than we know?

What is sex appeal?

While sex appeal is most often something divined only by the perceiver, something relating to their own personal preferences, there are some basic, physiological occurrences that may cause one person to exude more sex appeal than another.

Pheromones

Sexual attraction comes down to these hormones and how they affect people around them. Pheromones are believed to work as cue cards for reproduction. Studies have shown that the more pheromones released by a woman, the less her physical attractiveness matters to men. Women give off a pheromone during ovulation that has been found to raise testosterone levels in men. Humans have a special pit in their noses called a VNO that senses pheromones. In other words, the nose may be the ultimate erogenous zone.

Body Odour

Body odour has been reported to affect a female's choice of partner. Studies have shown that women are unlikely to sleep with a man if he doesn't 'smell right' to her. A study in Switzerland showed that women were most likely to be attracted by the smell of a man with a different immune system to hers. A child resulting from such a union would be most likely to have a better immune system and so be less susceptible to disease.

Symmetry

The better your physical symmetry, the better the other aspects of your physiology are likely to be, such as your brain, your immune system and, most importantly, your ability to reproduce. Although you may be unaware of it, when you find someone beautiful, you are most likely thinking of them as being symmetrical. It has been discovered that the more symmetrical a man's facial features, and the more symmetrical a woman's body, the more attractive their body odour is likely to be to a member of the opposite sex.

Into the mouth: Aphrodisiacs

There are many natural alternatives to Viagra, as these solutions for a dwindling sex life show. Picked from around the world, they will shock and surprise . . . and some should come with a health warning.

Food

According to ancient Chinese tradition, **APRICOTS** and **PEACHES** with their smooth soft skins and firm juicy flesh, are symbols of sensuality.

Iranians believe **TURNIPS** cooked in milk to be good for a dwindling sex life.

It is widely believed that **ASPARAGUS** has aphrodisiac powers. In France in the nineteenth century, a nervous bridegroom might be expected to eat several courses of it during the prenuptial dinner.

OYSTERS are perhaps the best known aphrodisiac, having a decidedly suggestive shape, texture and taste.

Montezuma, the sixteenth-century Aztec king, was said to drink fifty cups of **HOT CHOCOLATE** before entering his harem, for its qualities as an aphrodisiac.

Chocolate contains phenylethylamine (PEA), a natural substance said to cause a similar reaction in the body as that when you fall in love. It also contains the stimulants caffeine and theobromine.

Some people maintain that a mixture of equal parts of **sour cream** and **beer** is a powerful aphrodisiac.

The smells of **PUMPKIN PIE, LIQUORICE, BAKED CINNAMON BUNS, VANILLA, PIZZA** and **BUTTERED POPCORN** are reported to cause the greatest increase of blood flow to the penis.

According to the *Kama Sutra*, a mixture of **CLARIFIED BUTTER, HONEY, SUGAR, LIQUORICE, FENNEL** and **MILK** promotes sexual vigour.

GINSENG has long been used in many Asian countries as an aphrodisiac, and is said to work by increasing blood flow, which is associated with the heightened state of sexual excitement. It apparently improves sperm count.

A **TESTICLE** of a ram or goat boiled in **SUGARY MILK** and drunk is supposed to help out the male libido, according to the *Kama Sutra*.

Magical Aphrodisiacs

A dangerous concoction is suggested by the *Kama Sutra* as an aphrodisiac: mix powders of white thorn apple, long pepper and black pepper with honey and then anoint the penis. This is supposed to make a woman subject to a man's will. It is also a potent poison.

In parts of Scandinavia it is believed that a few drops of your blood mixed into someone's drink will cause them to desire you.

Cleopatra believed that drinking pearls dissolved in vinegar would make her more sexually desirable.

Persians ate pills of crushed pearls, rubies, gold dust and ambergris as an aphrodisiac.

LOVE SPELLS AND CHARMS

A Woman's Kissing Spell

Apply red lipstick to your lips and make a kiss print on a piece of white paper, then take a red candle and burn the paper while chanting, 'Kiss me when we meet, kiss me [insert person's full name], Greet me with your lips, and say you missed me. But most of all kiss me.' Make sure you have some water handy to keep the flames under control.

Visualise the person you want to kiss you, and think of love.

To Arouse a Lover's Interest

Mix four eggs, half a teaspoon of ginger, and a pinch of salt and pepper in a bowl. Fill half an eggshell with water twice, pouring it into the bowl. Beat and then cook the mixture in a frying pan. While still soft, trace your name at the top of the omelette and your lover's at the bottom. Fold it to the hide the words.

The omelette should be served with a salad of bananas, peaches and cherries and eaten by your lover.

To Make a Lover More Passionate in Bed

Write your lover's name on a red candle, stroke it nine times with musk oil and then pass it through the smoke of musk incense. Light the candle once a day, burning half an inch each time. When the candle is finished, wrap it in red satin and keep it under your bed for one month.

To Find a Lover

This spell is best done during the waxing moon, preferably on the first Friday after the new moon.

Light some jasmine incense and imagine a protective circle around yourself. Write down on a piece of paper all the qualities that you desire in a lover. Place a few drops of rose oil on a pink candle and say 'I consecrate and charge this candle as a magical tool for attracting love'.

Then light the candle and chant, 'Moon of love, shining bright, aid me in my spell tonight. Guide my true love to me, as I send so must it be.' Now picture yourself attracting a lover. Look at the candle flame and say three times, 'Hear me as I call above, come to me my one true love.' Your spell is complete.

To Increase Attractiveness to the Opposite Sex

Wear a peacock feather or an image of a peacock. For instance, you could wear a peacock feather pinned inside your clothes, or wear earrings shaped like peacocks. Look in the mirror and repeat, 'I am spreading my tail feathers.' When you leave the house, notice all the potential lovers out there. You will find an increase in the attention you receive.

To Discover if your Partner is your True Love

If you are not sure whether you and your partner are meant for each other, do this love spell. Take two pennies and toss them into the air saying, 'May we each go to our own true love.' Repeat this thirteen times. If you are right for each other, you will stay together, but if you are not meant for each other the relationship will not last much longer. You will both end up with your own true love eventually.

To Find True Love

Prepare a small mixture of rose, lavender, jasmine and ylang ylang oils and have two pink candles and nine rose petals ready. Then light some rose or lavender incense, take a pink candle and hold it in your hands. Visualise your desire to find true love. Grasping the candle at its midpoint with your left index finger and thumb, use your right index finger and thumb to stroke the mixture of essential oils on the candle. Repeat the process, using the other hand.

While holding the candle, visualise a pure white beam of light entering your body through the soles of your feet and another beam of white light coming down and entering your body through the top of your head. Picture the energy of these beams of light flowing through your body and reaching your hands, causing them to feel warm and to tingle. Now continue to stroke your candle until you feel the energy from your hands transfer to the candle. Your candle is now charged with your desire. Place it, still lit, in a candlestick.

Pick up the next pink candle and hold it in your hands. Visualise the person, or type of person you desire and anoint the candle as before.

Place the lit candles in holders and encircle them with the nine rose petals. Visualise yourself in a loving relationship with the perfect mate and allow your candles to burn down completely. Keep one of the rose petals to carry with you in your purse or pocket to reinforce your desire, and scatter the eight remaining petals to the four corners of the wind, as an offering.

FLIRTATIOUS FEASTS

Whether you eat the food you've prepared at home, or take it with you for a picnic, cooking for someone else is always romantic. The effort involved is impressive, particularly if you take care over presentation. Cooking with a partner is also fun – although you can become distracted!

Don't skimp on ingredients, and keep things simple. If you are taking the food on a picnic, take a nice quilt or a crisp white cloth to sit upon. Use real glasses, cutlery and plates.

Chocolate-covered Strawberries

Combining two sensual foods – strawberries and chocolate – this treat is easy to make, and melts easily in your mouth.

1 block of milk chocolate
Strawberries for two

Slowly warm the chocolate in a glass bowl over a saucepan filled with hot water. Stir continuously.

When the chocolate melts, dip in the strawberries. Drizzle the leftover chocolate over the cooling strawberries. Rest the fruit on waxed paper and chill for two hours. Eat.

You could also try this with skinned bananas and orange slices.

Coeurs à la Crème

A custard-based dessert for the heart, la coeur, and enough of a tradition that you can buy the moulds in speciality food shops.

For the base:

1 lb fromage frais
4 oz double cream

For the strawberry sauce:

1 pt of strawberries
3 tbsp granulated sugar
1 tbsp fresh lemon juice

Purée the fromage frais in a food processor for 30 seconds and whip the cream. Fold the two together.

Lay cheesecloth in the moulds, and pack the cheese mixture into them. Drain if necessary and leave to set in the refrigerator for 24 hours.

When set, tip the 'hearts' on to plates and peel off the cheesecloth.

Purée the ingredients for the strawberry sauce but do not strain. Pour it over the Coeurs à la Crème.

New Chilli Powder

Hot in more ways than one, this spice mixture should be used wherever cayenne or chilli pepper is called for. Contains cloves, a known Chinese aphrodisiac.

5 tbsp ground mild chilli peppers
2 tbsp dried oregano
1½ tbsp ground cumin
½ tsp chilli powder
1 tbsp dried cloves

Simply combine all the ingredients and toast in a skillet for two minutes.

Candied Apples

Apples have long been associated with both love and hedonism. Candied apples are bright red and tempting, and gloriously, sensually sticky.

4 medium red apples
4 wooden skewers
Waxed paper

For the caramel:
8 oz granulated sugar
4 fl oz water
3 oz corn syrup
2 inches of cinnamon stick
Red food colouring

Place the ingredients for the caramel in a saucepan. Boil without stirring for three minutes until the syrup reaches the soft-crack stage, when it solidifies if a little is dropped in cold water.

Set the pan of syrup over – not in – boiling water. Add four drops of red food colouring.

Working quickly, twirl the apples on their sticks in the mixture, and allow to cool on the waxed paper.

Asparagus with Orange and Hazelnuts

A sensual, aesthetic masterpiece with the long, firm asparagus and the round, hard hazelnuts. Oranges are ever associated with sex because of their secret insides and ready juices.

1 lb asparagus, bottoms snapped off
2 tbsp butter
1½ tbsp grated orange zest
6 oz chopped, toasted hazelnuts
Juice of half an orange

Roast, steam or boil the asparagus. Place a large skillet over medium heat and cook the rest of the ingredients until the butter is slightly browned. Then add the cooked asparagus and toss several times. Season to taste.

French Hot Chocolate

A rich, liquid confection; drink this instead of eating a dessert.

You will need:

1 cup single or double cream
8 oz plain or milk chocolate cut into small pieces
1 tsp vanilla or ½ tsp Kahlua or Grand Marnier
Ground nutmeg or cinnamon and whipped cream to decorate.

Bring the cream to the boil then immediately remove from heat and whisk in the chocolate. Strain the mixture in a tea strainer.

For each cup of chocolate stir together 2 ounces of above mixture with 2 ounces of milk, water or coffee. Heat through and stir in the vanilla or liqueur. Top with cream and sprinklings of nutmeg or cinnamon.

UNDER THE COVERS – IN THE BEDROOM

Feng Shui

Feng Shui is an ancient Chinese art relating to energy. Literally translated as 'wind and water', it is the doctrine of modifying your physical surroundings to enhance your luck and wellbeing. Experts believe that 'space clearing' (ridding the home of clutter) leads to a better sex life, possibly because of the relaxing nature of clear, organised surroundings.

In Feng Shui, the south-west corner of the home is particularly relevant in matters of love and requires special attention.

Crystals

For a night of passion, place a candle or a crystal in the south-west corner of your bedroom. This activates luck relating to love. The ideal crystal for this purpose is either a rose quartz or yellow citrine.

Mirrors

Remove all mirrors from the bedroom, as they represent a third party. The same goes for the television, which is also distracting.

The Bed

The bed should never be in front of the door, or one or both parties in a relationship will be sickly. Pink bed sheets raise positive energy that enhances feelings of love and romance.

Flowers

No dead or dried flowers should be near you at any time, as they create bad energy. Red roses should be avoided; as tokens of love they are supposed to bleed the relationship.

Birds

A picture of lovebirds in the south-west corner of the home helps romance to blossom.

A pair of china mandarin ducks in the south-west corner of the bedroom is conducive to love. Wooden ducks are not recommended. Place a vase with a fresh rose (not red) behind the ducks for more effective Feng Shui.

Hearts

A red heart in the south-west corner of the bedroom encourages love to enter a person's life.

Lighting

A chandelier (with candles or otherwise) in the south-west corner of a home is one way to stimulate romance. Soft lighting is encouraged as it leads to romantic feelings. Candles in all shapes and sizes are conducive to love. They enhance the home, as well as the possibility of romance.

Secret Recipe

The ultimate recipe to attract a lover: place clean, coloured pebbles inside a glass or crystal bowl, and fill with clear, fresh water. Float flower petals and candles on top. Light candles daily for a short period, and replace the petals and water immediately afterwards.

MASSAGE FOR LOVERS

Massage is one of the oldest forms of medical care. There are depictions of massage in Egyptian tomb paintings, and a Chinese medical text dating to 2700 BC describes its advantages.

The Greeks and Romans were also firm believers in its importance; Julius Caesar had a daily massage to treat neuralgia.

Easy to learn, fun to administer, and divine to receive, massage has unlimited benefits, from improved circulation to strengthening the immune system. Massage is also great for relationships – the physical contact and relaxation will generate a greater intimacy between you.

Massage oils are readily available from chemists and health food shops. You only need to use a tablespoon or so of massage oil, warmed in your hands. Never rush a massage of any sort, try not to use your nails and make sure you have skin contact with your lover at all times.

Body Massage

Start by having your partner lie face down, and straddle their hips.

Spread your fingers, keeping them stiff, and rake them down the back from shoulders to buttocks, and then across from the spine outwards.

Lift the body gently along the sides of the back and shoulders, pulling the skin up and then lowering gently.

Don't neglect the arms and hands: a gentle squeezing

along the limbs and a circling motion on the hands and fingers help to relax the entire body.

Spiral your thumbs firmly along the lower back from the crack of the buttocks outwards.

For the buttocks, use the gentle pressure of your entire fist. Start in the dimple on either side, and work inwards in a kneading motion.

Use a gentle grabbing, squeezing motion on the thighs, concentrating both hands on one thigh at a time.

Head and Neck Massage

Areas of the neck can be damaged if too much pressure is applied. Do not attempt to massage the front of the neck or the throat. Always ask your partner if they are comfortable.

Have your partner lie on their stomach, head facing to one side.

Having rubbed a small amount of massage oil into your hands, begin the massage by gently squeezing the neck between your thumb and fingers, using alternating hands.

Using your fingertips, make small circles up the spine towards the head.

Gently lift the head by the sides of the neck, letting it drop back down gently.

Holding the skin at the base of the head gently in one hand, push down on the shoulders using the other hand.

Keeping each hand in the same general location, gently probe with fingers to find tight muscles, which will feel like thick knots or bands under the skin.

Applying pressure, gently but firmly work the tight areas loose. Gently turn your partner's head, and repeat the above steps.

Wipe any excess oil from your hands, and begin rubbing your partner's scalp in small circles with fingertips, using extra care around the temples and the base of the skull.

Sweep fingers from the hairline to the top of the head, applying slight pressure.

Gently turn your partner's head, and repeat.

Foot Massage

Foot massage is deeply relaxing and a good alternative to a body massage if you have limited time or space. Reflexology is a more refined and thorough form of foot massage that is based on the principle that different parts of the foot have corresponding parts in the body.

Tending to the big toes, for example, will also treat the head. Treating the entire foot will have a therapeutic effect on the whole body.

Kneel in front of your partner's right foot. Your partner may be seated or lying down.

Having applied a small amount of lotion or oil to the hands, support the foot with both hands, stroking the top of the foot with your thumbs from the base of the toes to the ankle.

Support the foot in your right hand and use your left thumb and index finger to squeeze between the joints of each foot. Massage each digit individually, gently rolling, rubbing and squeezing the entire toe, including the nail. Carefully pull on each toe, stretching it slightly.

Rest your left hand on the top of the foot, and roll and press the knuckles of your right hand into the ball of the foot, repeating the action three times.

Still resting your left hand on top of the foot, stroke the heel of your right hand firmly down the ball of the foot and into the arch, and then down the heel, repeating three times.

Supporting the foot with the fingers of both hands, stroke both thumbs firmly up the sole.

At the ball of the foot, stroke out a T shape, and rub back down towards the heel. Repeat six times.

Sandwich the foot between your hands and stroke several times up towards the body.

Repeat all these steps with the other foot.

Hand Massage

Hand massage is great for those for those who work with computers and find their fingers and wrists aching at the end of the day. Best of all, it can be done almost anytime, anywhere.

Having worked some oil between your own hands, take your partner's hand and gently work circles into the back of the hand with your fingers, placing your thumb on the palm.

Gently pinch the webbing between the fingers of the hand between your thumb and middle finger.

Using both hands, 'fold' the hand by pressing thumbs into the palm and running finger firmly from the middle of the hand to the edges. Repeat several times, including the knuckles closest to the palm.

Press the tips of each finger, then work down each finger, gently rubbing between the joints. Pull each finger gently.

Aromatherapy for Romantics

Aromatherapy is the use of pure essential oils from fragrant plants to help improve the quality of life and address health problems. It is part of phytotherapy – the science of using the whole plants or parts of plants for medicinal purposes.

Though aromatherapy is relatively new to the United Kingdom, it has been used for thousands of years in other parts of the world. Ancient Egyptians used essential oils in cosmetics and in embalming. The modern practice of aromatherapy developed primarily in twentieth-century Europe.

Jasmine is believed to be the greatest floral aphrodisiac of all, and has been used at least since the time of Cleopatra for seduction. It is one of many white, night blooming flowers known to have this quality. All these flowers contain indole, part of the odour of putrefaction.

The Oils

Rose oil is for love, and is believed to open the hearts of both men and women.

Sandalwood is another aphrodisiac, and sets the tone for the sharing and fulfilling of fantasies.

Ylang Ylang is a sweet and exotic oil, with soothing and aphrodisiac qualities.

Lavender is a restorative oil that balances the mind and spirit. It calms or stimulates, according to the needs of the body.

Myrrh is not strictly an essential oil, but the resin from a tree. Widely used as incense, it has a mysterious and meditative scent.

Clary Sage is an uplifting oil that induces feelings of wellbeing and balance.

Patchouli is a musky oil, used to scent linen in the East, and for its sensual qualities.

In aromatherapy, essential oils are used in two ways: inhaled or applied to the skin.

Inhaling Essential Oils

When inhaled, the molecules of the oils are believed to stimulate the nose's olfactory nerve, sending messages to the brain's limbic system – the part controlling memory and emotion. Scientists believe stimulation of the limbic system can effect other bodily systems, such as the nervous system and the immune system.

Inhalation of essential oils can also impact the respiratory system directly. Anyone who has ever had a cold knows the effects of inhaling eucalyptus, which may help clear the sinuses.

The simplest way to inhale an essential oil is to sniff the undiluted oil itself. (You should not get the liquid into your nose. Some of the oils may irritate the skin if undiluted.)

Other inhalation mixtures include:

Oil diluted in mineral oil such as in a bubble bath or perfume.

Spray. About three drops of oil can be added to water in a spray bottle, and the spray can be used like an air freshener.

The oil can be used in an oil diffuser. A diffuser is a small stove with a candle or other heat source on the bottom and a small well of water on top. Oil added to the water will disperse as the oil heats, scenting the air. About six drops of oil are recommended.

A few drops of a relaxing oil like lavender can be sprinkled on a pillow as a sleep aid.

Some candles are made with essential oils. Burning the candle will disperse the scent.

Applying Oils to Your Skin

Applying essential oils to the skin causes them to be absorbed into the body. Some oils have recognisable physical effects, such as assisting the reduction of swelling. Others are used mostly for their psychological value and may help promote things like relaxation and invigoration. Make sure that you know which oils must avoid contact with the skin.

Always dilute the essential oil first before applying it to the skin. Often a 'carrier' oil is used as the diluting agent. A carrier oil is a pure, unscented oil such as soybean, almond or mineral oil. Synthetic oils may interfere with the scent of the essential oil. This combined oil can now be applied through massage, or as a moisturiser or perfume. About two to three parts oil should be added to every 100 parts of the carrier. For sensitive skin, halve the amount of essential oil.

Other means of applying the oils to the skin include:

A compress. Mix your oil with water, and dip a cloth into the mixture. Use the cloth as a compress.

The oil can be added to a warm bath. Minimum advised soaking time is fifteen minutes. About six drops of oil are usually recommended per bath.

The oil can be added to an unperfumed, non-synthetic cream as a moisturiser. As with the carrier oil, about two to three parts of essential oil should be added to every 100 parts of the cream or lotion. People with sensitive skin should halve the amount of essential oil.

DREAMS AND THEIR DIVINATION

People have always been fascinated by dreams and their interpretation. Freud most famously thought dreams (as well as almost every other human function) were concerned with repressed desire. The following is a list of interpretations of some themes that may occur in your dreams.

Adultery

Dreaming of adultery signifies that you are seeking outer sustenance instead of looking within for answers. It indicates an integration of the male and female parts of self.

Breasts

This is not a sexual dream, but about being wholly accepted for oneself.

Buttocks

Dreaming about buttocks is an instruction to the dreamer to stop, sit down and consider their current situation.

Chocolate

Chocolate represents a need for approval, or the deserving of a treat for a job well done.

Contraception

This can be either a positive or negative dream. It can indicate a measure used to prevent the self from moving in unwanted directions, or a cutting off of creative power.

Cupid

Dreaming of Cupid should encourage the dreamer to start taking some romantic risks, and promises a positive outcome to blossoming love affairs.

Erotic

An erotic dream asks the dreamer to be more attentive to the body's sexual needs, and to listen to the libido.

Feast

A big celebration reminding the dreamer they have done something well.

Genitals

Genitalia represent creative or sexual energy, or a source of illusion. A call to question one's sexual identity.

Heart

If you dream about cutting out a heart, you need to be more open to feelings. If you are being stabbed in the heart you are giving too much to others who don't necessarily appreciate your compassion. Hearts are generally a sign of spiritual and emotional love.

Homosexuality

If you dream about having sex with a known person, the dream is about integrating their qualities into yourself. It may also be a dream about your own sexuality.

Impotence

Dreaming of impotence signifies suppression, a fear of one's own power. Stop taking yourself so seriously.

Incest

This indicates a merging of different parts of self. All persons in the dream are you – this is not a sexual dream.

Kiss

A kiss symbolises warmth and affection or the beginnings of new love. However, beware the kiss of betrayal.

Love

To dream of love is to dream of the depths within yourself.

Lover

Dreaming of a lover indicates a desire for warmth, love and affection and the integration of the male and female parts of self.

Masturbation

This represents the need for physical and emotional release.

Nude

Dreaming of nakedness means that you are totally open and exposed, not hiding who and what you are.

Orgasm

This tells the dreamer they are not having enough sexual contact in waking life.

Orgy

This is a warning against over-indulgence, and of allowing energy to spread in too many directions. A recommendation to rest.

Prostitution

To dream of prostitution shows that you are misusing energy to get what you think you want. It is a calling to be true to the self.

Sensual

A sensual dream is a call to get in touch with your own sexuality. More physical contact is necessary for a healthy inner life.

Sexual Intercourse

Dreaming of sex indicates a merger of the various aspects of self. If the dream is of having sex with someone you know, it suggests that you wish to take on some of their characteristics.

Underwear

To dream of undergarments means that you are hiding from part of your true self.

ALL IN THE LOCATION

– Places of Passion, Romantic Retreats and Hedonistic Holidays

Holidays are a great way of meeting new people and whether it's a holiday fling you're looking for, or a potential mate for life after exhausting your local resources, you're sure to find something. If you are already a couple, spending time just the two of you with no bills or deadlines to worry about will allow time for you to relax in each other's company again. If it's hedonism you're after, your anonymity combined with being away from home, should allow your excess-loving side to reach even greater heights.

Places of Passion

While the most important thing about sex should be the person you are doing it with, the location can turn a standard session into an unforgettable experience. Forget sand in those hard to reach places or rolling around in mud and leaves – these are the crème de la crème of sexy places.

New Orleans

New Orleans is famous for consuming libidinous tourists, only to spit them out days later, hung over and happy. It starts with the city's French origins, and it ends with the city's jazz – its pride and its creation. Jazz is by its nature sexy, and it arose from the sensuality long propagated by the city's vast red-light district and proud gambling tradition. New Orleans is a port town and so it specialises in sailors; folk who rarely stand to be lonely long. New Orleans is also famous for its dark bourbon, as well as a superstitious fear of the voodoo brought by immigrants and honed in an atmosphere of slavery and mistrust.

The elements blend to create the sensuality and irresistible darkness of New Orleans.

The Mile High Club

The most famous of flying clubs meets in an aeroplane, the party beginning a mile or more up in the skies soon after the seat-belt light goes out. The aim of the revellers is sex and the excitement provided by the forbidden and the novelty of the location, makes for a memorable experience. The most frequently chosen venue is the plane's toilet but other options are to utilise the airline issued blankets, and snuggle up with a loved one when the lights are dimmed. The first-class enclosed berths offered by some carriers provide a luxurious alternative.

'Sandals'

Palm trees, bright sunlight, endless beaches of white sands, cocktails served in coconut shells . . . this is Sandals, a series of all-inclusive resorts devoted to couples: no children, no singles. Located in heavenly places such as Jamaica, Antigua, St Lucia and the Bahamas, the resorts also organise 'WeddingMoons' that combine the wedding and honeymoon into one tight package. For the hedonist who loves luxury, being pampered and decadence, this is the perfect hedonistic holiday.

Romantic Retreats

Like good sex, good romance is subjective. Some may think a ride across the desert on the back of a Harley is romantic, while others will settle for a night of Chinese take-away and Tsing-Tao beer. The best bet for a romantic getaway is to discover a partner's most decadent fantasy, and follow it.

Health Farms

Luxuriate in deep mud baths, cuddle up together in fluffy towels, and enjoy plenty of fresh healthy food and exercise. Your improved complexion and toned bodies can only add to the romance already in your life, kindling a glowing flame to a roaring fire. Health farms can be attended alone, in groups or with a partner. The advantage of going with a partner is obvious: after a day of being massaged, oiled, pampered and otherwise beautified, it would be a fine luxury to snuggle away in a private room with the one you love.

Rome

There is something in the air in Rome that is compellingly erotic. People return from the ancient city reporting the air to be sepia-coloured.

Rome is also incurably romantic. One of the gods of the city, Angerina, is always depicted with a gag in her mouth to ensure she won't reveal the secret name of the city – Roma spelt backwards, or Amor. Rome gained her vast empire through brilliant military planning, and she has kept her city undiminished through the millennia with promises of Amor.

Log Cabins

Imagine the Christmas card image; the sheepskin rug in front of the roaring fire, the bottle of warming red wine, the snowdrifts outside and a huge double bed covered in soft blankets to fall into at midnight. The cabin has to be cold enough to get away with a fire, and far enough from the road to give a feeling of absolute intimacy. The idea can either be to wander around in the woods showing off each other's nature skills, or to simply curl up in the luxury of seclusion.

Hot-air Ballooning

Romantic on the face of it, hot-air ballooning is in fact cold, and involves entertaining a third person – the man keeping you aloft. Still, the world is much more beautiful and peaceful from a height, and ballooning is quieter than almost any other sort of flying. Package tours often include a luxury champagne picnic.

Paris

Paris has long been said to have the most beautiful women, the best wine and the greatest bounty of excellent food. The ancient feel of the place, and the sensual nature of its architecture combine to create an aura of romance.

The route along the river is perfect for sated lovers walking home to their hotel room.

Couple all this with the French accent and there can be little wonder as to why people believe they fall in love first with Paris, and then with the person who brought them there.

Venice

Venice, is often called the most romantic city.

Perhaps it's the water, in itself sensuous. The city is filled with artists and musicians with beautiful voices who are always available for hire to serenade a loved one. Venice, to the outside world, has a sense of slow paced sensuality, underlined by the innovative acceptance of watery roads and buildings standing long where few would have thought to build. The birthplace of Casanova and once the home of some of the world's most famous courtesans – professional lovers for those who could pay – Venice remains invested in sensuality.

Hedonistic Holidays

Hedonists, with their general philosophy of living a life of pleasure without regard to consequences, are generally not well received in large quantities. However, hedonism is also about self-indulgence, which can range from splashing out on an expensive bottle of champagne to going that bit further and hiring someone to feed it to you.

The Orient Express

An expensive way to impress, but worth it. A trip can last anywhere from a few days to a few weeks, and the trains travel through such diverse places as Bath, Budapest, and Brisbane. Described by many as a five-star hotel on wheels with Regency-style furniture and trimmings, glamorous en suite rooms and superb food, the Orient Express is the ultimate in luxurious travel.

Amsterdam

Amsterdam has been attracting lovers and hedonists since its popularity as a trading post in the thirteenth century when sailors would dock to find spiritual sustenance in the beautiful churches, and physical fulfilment in the arms of prostitutes. A trip to Amsterdam is incomplete without a visit to the world famous red-light district where women in leather and lace press provocatively against full-length windows. Less extreme is to relax with a smoke in the Vondelpark, read home-published erotic poetry or have a neck massage. Later, you can sample the strong Dutch beer and the many varieties of marijuana listed on café menus. Amsterdam's refreshingly liberal 'live and let live' attitude will suit the most dedicated of pleasure seekers, where everything conspires to create a charged atmosphere of sensuality.

Monte Carlo

This warm Mediterranean city has the best sort of hedonist – the rich sort. Gambling has long been the preserve of the true hedonist, and for the wealthy attempting to prove their devil-may-care attitude, this is the place to be. Along with high stakes tables, Monte Carlo has sun and water, and with that combination come yachts, beautiful girls and alcohol. Truly, Monte Carlo is a temple of hedonism – as long as you can afford it.

Las Vegas

Las Vegas is for the lucky hedonist on a budget. Unique among most other tourist destinations, travellers try to reach the city's famous strip at night, when the pure tacky essence is most obvious, and lined up for all to see. For those who gamble, drinks are free all night. For those who gamble high, the bed is free, as is breakfast. It's the best sort of city for a person not looking for love – one that seduces for the sole purpose of using its lovers. Nevada remains one of the few places in the New World where keeping company with a prostitute doesn't mean getting arrested.

A Night at the Opera

Have a luxurious weekend away at a city with a grand opera house. Opera is renowned for being indolent, opulent and lush. The voices are big, the seats are velvet and you dress up to go. Choose a lavish opera such as La Bohème or La Traviata, but avoid operas with comprehensive librettos or projected subtitles – the mystery of what they're singing is part of the allure.

Ibiza

The perfect place for a hedonist, the holiday resorts on the island of Ibiza are typically packed with enough people to make for a guilt-free holiday. Most unions and excesses will only be witnessed by people who don't care. All visitors are actively encouraged to drink and dance all night, and to make every effort to encourage other people to join them. Make your time in Ibiza as debauched and dirty as you can . . . before returning home with embarrassing photos to jog your hazy, alcohol-steeped memory.

Hedonism I, II and III

The name says it all. These resorts are all located in warm places (Jamaica and the Bahamas) for the specific purpose of allowing people to walk around in the nude. Unlike nudist resorts however, lust is not discouraged. Like Ibiza, the general flavour is that of drinking, dancing and singing all night – then sleeping it off in a hammock on the beach.

THE WEIRD AND THE WONDERFUL

You won't believe your eyes when you read this selection of the strangest tales of sex, love and hedonism from around the world. Not for the faint-hearted . . .

SEX

Bathing Beauties

The Moorish baths offered a service whereby women would pull out clumps of men's pubic hair to induce orgasms.

Bzzz . . .

Cleopatra is said to have had a box with bees trapped inside that she would place against her genitals as a vibrator.

Love Is A Many Splintered Thing

Dendrophilia is the term used to describe those who have a sexual fixation on trees. In some cultures men would even marry trees.

Hot But Not Cross

Early Christians were often reluctant to give up the Roman tradition of phallus worship and continued to bake bread in the shape of sex organs. Finally the church capitulated and said the bread could be baked on Christian holidays providing they were marked with a cross. The result? Hot cross buns.

Work and Play

The Code of Jewish Law regulates sexual performance according to a husband's profession: 'Men of a strong constitution who enjoy the pleasures of life, having profitable pursuits at home and are tax-exempt should perform their marital duty nightly.

Labourers who work in the town where they reside should perform their marital duty twice weekly; but if they are employed in another town, only once a week. Men who convey freight on camels from distant places should attend to their marital duty once in thirty days.'

LOVE

Oriental Gift Wrapping

In eighth-century Japan aristocrats practised the art of Tsutsami. They would wrap their genitals in silk and ribbons in complex designs and then offer them as gifts to their lovers.

You Drive Me Crazy

President Franklin D. Roosevelt is reported to have had a long affair with his female chauffeur. It was she who sat in vigil by his deathbed instead of his wife, Eleanor.

Eleanor was herself documented to have had an affair with a female journalist.

E(a)rotic

Legend has it that Van Gogh cut off his ear and sent it to a lover as a token of his unrequited affection. Actually, Van Gogh sliced off only part of his earlobe after a fight with Gauguin and took the piece to a brothel hoping to find the artist there. When he couldn't find his friend he gave the piece to a prostitute. History does not tell us what he hoped Gauguin's reaction would be to the fleshy particle.

HEDONISM

Roman Regurgitation

In ancient Rome it was common practice among the elite to dine in a room called the vomitorium. In this room men would feast upon the rich and exotic delicacies served.

When a man felt full he would have a servant tickle the back of his neck to cause him to vomit. Having created the necessary room in his stomach, he would resume feasting.

Shoes, Glorious Shoes

Imelda Marcos is best known to the outside world for the 1,200 pairs of shoes she left behind at Malacanang Palace in the Philippines after fleeing with her husband, President Ferdinand Marcos, in the political uprising of 1986.

They are now on display in the palace's museum, which even sells postcards of them.

The Mad Monks of Medmenham

Sir Francis Dashwood, the Chancellor of the Exchequer from 1761–2, led the Hellfire Club at Medmenham Abbey near the Thames in the eighteenth century. Members congregated once or twice a week to devote their time to black magic rites, and meetings were held in a temple with an entrance formed to resemble a vagina.

ASTROLOGICAL SEX, LOVE AND HEDONISM

Aries

March 21 – April 20

The Lover:

Dynamic, thrill-seeking and leaders of charmed lives, Aries' are adventurers who require little persuasion to do anything.

The Date:

Activity dates are best for people born under the sign of restless Aries, with dancing, bowling, rock-climbing and golf all being good suggestions. Fast foods or spicy dishes are good bets at mealtimes.

The Drink:

Hot and Creamy

Mix one shot of Aftershock Cinnamon Liqueur and a dash of raspberry schnapps into a glass and fill to the top with pineapple juice.

Most Compatible:

Leo, Sagittarius.

Unlikely Match:

Cancer, Libra, Capricorn, Aries.

Taurus

April 21 – May 20

The Lover:

People under this sign will eat a lot, drink a lot and love a lot, but only in private and only with one special person.

The Date:

Given to decadence at home, indulgent Taureans should be served a rich dinner and taken on a romantic stroll to finish off the evening. Picnics are a good option, or a cosy night in front of a warm fire.

The Drink:

Buttery Nipple

A shot made up of equal parts sambuca and butterscotch schnapps.

Most Compatible:

Virgo, Capricorn.

Unlikely Match:

Aquarius, Leo, Scorpio.

Gemini

May 21 – June 20

The Lover:

Gemini is the unpredictable sign of the zodiac: erratic and striving. Drinking is the order of the day, and variety is the spice of life.

The Date:

Easily bored, Gemini needs to be entertained by doing two things at once. Go to a yoga class in Las Vegas. Fly a kite while salsa dancing. Throw a wild party at a library.

The Drink:

Illicit Affair

Mix one shot of Irish Cream and a dash of peppermint schnapps into a shot glass and top with whipped cream.

Most Compatible:

Libra, Aquarius, Gemini.

Unlikely Match:

Virgo, Sagittarius, Pisces.

Cancer

June 21 – July 20

The Lover:

The homebodies of the zodiac are emotional and need security. Cancerians will be strong and loyal but you need to earn their trust first.

The Date:

Take things slowly with a Cancerian. Make a nice meal at home and rent a good film.
Take a telescope and go stargazing. Tell each other fairy tales.

The Drink:

Slow Comfortable Screw Up Against a Wall

Mix equal measures of vodka, sloe gin and Southern Comfort in a glass, fill to the top with orange juice and add a splash of Galliano.

Most Compatible:

Scorpio, Pisces.

Unlikely Match:

Libra, Capricorn, Aquarius, Cancer.

Leo

July 21 – August 20

The Lover:

If it's not money, it's affluence. Superstar Leo likes to be dined even more than being wined, and will eat it if it looks exotic or expensive – preferably both.

The Date:

Whatever you do with the lion, make sure it's impressive. Involve champagne, expensive flowers and strappy sandals. Whatever you talk about, make out you are an authority.

The Drink:

Morning Kiss

Pour a shot of apricot brandy and a shot of gin into a champagne glass and fill with champagne and orange juice.

Most Compatible:

Sagittarius, Aries.

Unlikely Match:

Scorpio, Aquarius, Taurus.

Virgo

August 21 – September 20

The Lover:

Virgos are often cautious perfectionists. Easily distracted and needing an excess of stimulation, Virgos are practical types who are hopeless with money.

The Date:

Whatever you do with a Virgo, keep it simple and keep it moving. Rollerskate in the park with a bag of bread to feed the ducks. Go to a museum attached to a botanical garden.

Visit a miniature golf course with a bar. Go on a walking tour around the city and know where there's a good restaurant serving ordinary food.

The Drink:

Get Laid
Mix one shot of vodka and a dash of raspberry schnapps in a glass and fill to the top with pineapple juice.

Most Compatible:

Capricorn, Taurus, Virgo.

Unlikely Match:

Sagittarius, Pisces, Gemini.

Libra

September 21 – October 20

The Lover:

Mellow Librans like to be seduced. They can be persuaded into hedonistic acts, but only in intimate groups.

The Date:

This sign is classy; heed the call of art and take a Libran for a date in a gallery, to the ballet or a poetry reading. Given to the occasional decadence, dessert dates might be considered, bypassing dinner all together. Aerial activities like kite flying and ballooning would also be popular.

The Drink:

Lady Love Fizz

Take two shots of gin, a few splashes of single cream, a dash of powdered sugar, juice of half a lemon and one egg white. Mix over ice and strain into a cocktail glass. Fill to the brim with sparkling water.

Most Compatible:

Aquarius, Gemini, Libra.

Unlikely Match:

Capricorn, Aries, Cancer.

Scorpio

October 21 – November 20

The Lover:

Scorpio is the ultimate wild child in the zodiac. Passionate and secretive, Scorpios are aware of limits, but don't see why they should pertain to them.

The Date:

Do something active with the dangerous, sexy Scorpion. Fly to a foreign country, go to the fair, sing badly in front of loads of people. Go to a party wearing the best costume.

The Drink:

Fast Freddie

One shot of Southern Comfort, one shot of Blue Hawaiian Maui schnapps, two shots of cranberry juice.

Most Compatible:

Pisces, Cancer.

Unlikely Match:

Aquarius, Taurus, Leo, Scorpio.

Sagittarius

November 21 – December 20

The Lover:

If you haven't done it yet, it's a Sagittarian who is likely to introduce you to it. Adventurous and blessed with boundless enthusiasm, Sagittarius thrives on challenge.

The Date:

Sagittarians like to be surprised, but in an ordinary fashion. Outdoorsy things like canoeing and camping go down well, and a visit to the zoo would not go amiss. Take a

Sagittarian, fishing or for a ride on the back of a big motorbike.

The Drink:

Frigid Hairy Virgin

Two shots of rum, one shot of Triple Sec, two shots of pineapple juice.

Most Compatible:

Aries, Leo.

Unlikely Match:

Pisces, Gemini, Virgo.

Capricorn

December 21 – January 20

The Lover:

Don't let their domestic exteriors fool you – once you get a Capricorn going it's almost impossible to stop them. They are given to wild bursts they'd rather not discuss later.

The Date:

The traditional Capricorn will appreciate a long limousine drive with champagne to a live music venue. They may well know how to ballroom dance, and have membership to a swanky bar or country club.

The Drink:

Arise My Love

A glass of chilled champagne with a dash of Creme de Menthe Green sunk at the bottom.

Most Compatible:

Taurus, Virgo.

Unlikely Match:

Aries, Cancer, Libra.

Aquarius

January 21 – February 20

The Lover:

Aquarians are inventive, eccentric and independent. They don't form deep relationships easily. They will eat, drink and be merry in great quantities, and with a large number of people.

The Date:

Whatever you do with the free spirit of the zodiac, make sure it's original. Meet up at midnight to go skinny-dipping. Try skydiving, snowboarding or bungee jumping. Eat weird food at a far away restaurant. Go fishing at dawn.

The Drink:

Run and Go Naked

Plenty of vodka, twelve cans of lager, two litres of old-fashioned lemonade. Pour into a big vat and serve at a party in plastic cups.

Most Compatible:

Gemini, Libra, Aquarius.

Unlikely Match:

Taurus, Leo, Scorpio.

Pisces

February 21 – March 20

The Lover:

Pisces are the dreamers of the zodiac. They are often enjoy fantasising, are wild in bed and fond of exotic outside locations.

The Date:

The original water babies might like to go sailing or visit an aquarium. A visit to the beach might be in order, or take them for a turn around an ice rink.

Foreign films, live music or a book reading may capture the imagination of a Piscean.

The Drink:

Sex in a Bubble Gum Factory

A shot of banana liqueur, a shot of Caracao Blue, a shot of apricot brandy and a shot of rum. Mix into a glass and fill to the top with lemonade.

Most Compatible:

Cancer, Scorpio, Pisces.

Unlikely Match:

Gemini, Virgo, Sagittarius.

. . . IN A NUTSHELL . . .

Room for Improvement

In today's society it is easy to be simply too busy to practise the fine art of seduction or take time out to indulge in hedonistic acts. The following ideas are designed to be quick-fix solutions that should inspire you to improve your life in those important areas.

Tips for lovers . . .

BLINDFOLD YOUR LOVER WITH AN ITEM OF CLOTHING YOU HAVE BEEN WEARING ALL DAY, AND LET THEM EXPLORE YOUR BODY.

RUN THE WISPS OF A FEATHER OVER YOUR LOVER'S BODY TO SEND THEM INTO SQUIRMING ECSTASY.

HANG A LARGE MIRROR ABOVE THE BED, OR MIRROR ONE WALL OF THE BEDROOM SO YOU WON'T MISS A THING.

ROLE-PLAY COMPLETE WITH PROPS AND COSTUMES.

MAKE A BOOK OF HANDWRITTEN FANTASIES TO SHARE WITH YOUR LOVER.

INVEST IN PASTEL LIGHT BULBS FOR THE BEDROOM, AND DRAPE LAMPS WITH GAUZY FABRIC. COLOURED LIGHTS DISTRACT FROM AND DIMINISH ANY BODILY IMPERFECTIONS.

SPRINKLE A FEW DROPS OF YOUR LOVER'S FAVOURITE FRAGRANCE ON A WARM LIGHT BULB OR RADIATOR TO DIFFUSE THE SCENT AROUND THE HOUSE.

LEARN HOW TO GIVE A GREAT MASSAGE.

WASH AND DRY SHEETS WITH A SPLASH OF YOUR PERFUME.

HAVE FUN TOGETHER IN THE BATH OR SHOWER WITH COLOURED BODY PAINTS.

INVEST IN WHIPPED CREAM, CHOCOLATE SAUCE . . . AND CHERRIES.

SHOWER TOGETHER EVERY DAY BEFORE WORK.

Tips for romantics . . .

SEND YOUR LOVER OFF TO WORK WITH A NOTE IN THEIR POCKET TELLING THEM HOW MUCH YOU LOVE THEM, OR WRITE A LOVE POEM FOR THEM. USE UNLINED PAPER AND A THICK FOUNTAIN PEN.

PLAN A SURPRISE WEEKEND AWAY, AND DON'T TELL ANY OF YOUR FRIENDS OR FAMILY WHERE IT IS. SECLUDED COTTAGES ARE A GOOD CHOICE IF YOU ARE WILLING TO COOK. A HOTEL MAY BE A BETTER CHOICE IF YOU WANT ROOM SERVICE OR ACCESS TO GOOD RESTAURANTS.

SPRINKLE ROSE PETALS OVER YOUR LOVER'S BED, SPELLING OUT THEIR NAME WITH FLOWERS.

ALWAYS SEND FLOWERS THE MORNING AFTER THE FIRST DATE, REGARDLESS OF YOUR SEX. DISCOVER YOUR PARTNER'S FAVOURITE FLOWER.

KEEP YOUR LARDER STOCKED WITH FOOD THAT CAN EASILY BE CONSUMED IN BED USING ONLY FINGERS. CHOCOLATE IS A GOOD CHOICE, AS ARE A VARIETY OF NUTS AND SMALL CHEESES. ITEMS THAT DO NOT CREATE CRUMBS ARE PREFERABLE.

READ ROMANTIC LITERATURE TO EACH OTHER. THE PASSAGES CAN BE PROSE OR POETRY, NEW OR OLD.

TREAT THE MOST IMPORTANT PERSON IN YOUR LIFE LIKE THE MOST IMPORTANT PERSON IN YOUR LIFE.

ALWAYS TELL YOUR PARTNER YOU LOVE THEM BEFORE YOU FALL ASLEEP, EVEN IF YOU'RE ANGRY.

EAT GARLIC AND ONIONS TOGETHER, NEVER ALONE.

LEARN TO COOK THE FOOD YOUR PARTNER LOVES BEST, AND THEN MAKE IT FOR THEM ONCE A MONTH.

Tips for hedonists . . .

MAKE LOVE OUTSIDE IN THE MIDDLE OF THE DAY. KEEP YOUR SHOES ON IN CASE YOU HAVE TO RUN.

RAVISH YOUR LOVER IN A DESERTED CORNER OF A CASTLE DURING A GUIDED TOUR.

BUY YOUR BELOVED A PAINTING INSTEAD OF PAYING THE RENT.

DRINK AN ENTIRE BOTTLE OF CHAMPAGNE WHILE SOAKING IN A BUBBLE BATH.

PARTY THROUGH AN ENTIRE WEEKEND.

SLEEP THROUGH AN ENTIRE WEEKEND.

SWIM NAKED IN A HOTEL POOL AFTER MIDNIGHT.

HAVE SEX IN THE BACK SEAT OF YOUR CAR EVEN WHEN THERE ARE OTHER PLACES YOU COULD GO.

SO **SEXY,**
REALLY **ROMANTIC**
AND THE **HEIGHTS**
OF **HEDONISM**

Dare to be inspired by these instances of sex, love and hedonism from the depths of history and the ranks of the rich and famous.

So Sexy

Marilyn Monroe singing 'Happy Birthday, Mr President' to John F. Kennedy. She had to be sewn into her white gown covered with crystals. The dress was so light and gauzy that it fitted into the palm of her hand.

The nude picture of John Lennon wrapped around Yoko Ono, gently kissing her cheek.

KING DAVID watching BATHSHEBA as she bathed on the roof. David later ensured Bathsheba's husband would be killed in battle so he could have her for himself.

On screen chemistry between MICKEY ROURKE and KIM BASINGER in 9½ Weeks.

Rocker Tommy Lee licking Pamela Anderson's face as a greeting when they first met.

Eve giving Adam the apple, giving rise to all the sex, love and hedonism ever since.

Really Romantic

Lady and the Tramp sharing a plate of spaghetti behind Tony's Restaurant in the film *Lady and the Tramp*.

Shah Jahan building the Taj Mahal as a mausoleum for his wife Mimtaz Mahal. Upon her death in childbirth, after bearing him thirteen children, Jahan built the structure as a monument to his eternal love.

CLARK GABLE and CAROLE LOMBARD – although a famous actor and comedy actress, they married and settled in domestic bliss in a farmhouse, calling each other Ma and Pa, and when they quarrelled he sent her doves in reconciliation.

EDWARD WINDSOR sacrificing his throne to be with WALLIS SIMPSON.

Joe DiMaggio, ex-husband to Marilyn Monroe, sent roses to her grave three times a week for twenty years after her death.

Sir Lancelot betraying King Arthur for the love of Guinevere.

Heights of Hedonism

ELVIS PRESLEY flying his daughter, a young LISA MARIE, to the Rocky Mountains for two hours so she could play in the snow, then flying her back home.

MARILYN MONROE pouring quantities of Chanel No. 5 into her bath water.

MICHAEL JACKSON purchasing a plane for the sole use of his chimpanzee.

The Roman emperor HADRIAN erecting sculptures of his lover ANTINOUS all over the Empire and declaring him a god.

GUNTHER SACHS courting BRIGITTE BARDOT by flying over her house in a helicopter, showering her home with roses.

RICHARD BURTON's gift to ELIZABETH TAYLOR – the 33.6-carat Krupp diamond.

WIT AND WISDOM: QUOTATIONS

Sex

Chastity: The most unnatural of all sexual perversions.

Aldous Huxley

Don't knock masturbation. It's sex with someone I love.

Woody Allen

My reaction to porno films is as follows: After the first ten minutes, I want to go home and screw. After the first twenty minutes, I never want to screw again as long as I live.

Erica Jong

Her breasts were apocalyptic – they would topple empires before they withered.

Richard Burton on Elizabeth Taylor

A promiscuous person is someone who is getting more than you are.

Victor Lownes

Sex: The pleasure is momentary, the position is ridiculous, and the expense is damnable.

Lord Chesterfield

I am as pure as the driven slush.

Tallulah Bankhead

Marriage has many pains, but celibacy has no pleasures.

Samuel Johnson

My notches fit her nooks.

Tom Hanks on wife Rita Wilson

Kissing don't last; cookery do!

George Meredith

We were always great in bed, the trouble usually started on the way to the bidet.

Ava Gardner on Frank Sinatra

Sex has become one of the most discussed subjects of modern times. The Victorians pretended it did not exist; the moderns pretend nothing else exists.

Fulton J. Sheen

Love

Life has taught us that love does not consist in gazing at each other but in looking outward together in the same direction.

Saint Exupery

A kiss is a lovely trick designed by nature to stop speech when words become superfluous.

Ingrid Bergman

There is no disguise which can hide love for long where it exists, or simulate it where it does not.

La Rochefoucauld

If you would be loved, love and be lovable.

Benjamin Franklin

Love is like the measles. We all have to go through it.

Jerome K. Jerome

The heart has its reasons which reason knows nothing of.

Blaise Pascal

Love and Scandal are the best sweeteners of tea.

Henry Fielding

Hedonism

Mad, bad and dangerous to know.

Charlotte Lamb of Lord Byron

Bigamy is having one wife too many. Monogamy is the same.

Oscar Wilde

Once, during Prohibition, I was forced to live for days on nothing but food and water.

W. C. Fields

Immorality: The morality of those who are having a better time.

H. L. Mencken

One can drink too much, but one can never drink enough.

Gotthold Ephraim Lessing

Between two evils I'll always pick the one I haven't tried before.

Mae West

One more drink and I'll be under my host.

Dorothy Parker

Music and women I cannot but give way to, whatever my business is.

Samuel Pepys

Man, being reasonable, must get drunk; the best in life is but intoxication.

George Noel Gordon

Pleasure's a sin, and sometimes sin's a pleasure.

Lord Byron

And painful pleasure turns to pleasing pain.

Edmund Spenser

THE A-Z OF SEX, LOVE AND HEDONISM

A

is for alcohol. Champagne for lovers, red wine for romantics and anything goes for a hedonist.

B

is for books. Books can tell you all you need to know about the history of the pleasures of the flesh, as well as inspiring you with new ideas.

C

is for chocolate, a sexy, indulgent treat, releasing serotonin, the feel-good hormone.

D

is for dancing. Choose a dance to suit your mood; sexy salsa, slow cheek-to-cheek, or wild clubbing.

E

is for explicit exhibitionism, exciting eroticism, and ecstasy.

F

is for foreplay. Foreplay can last all day, from saucy e-mailing during office hours to playing footsie over dinner . . . until the real fun starts when you have the evening to yourselves.

G

is for games; drinking games, sexual teases, stripteases, guessing games, surprises. Make sure you play with forfeits and prizes.

H

is for hangover. It is difficult to indulge in hedonism of the alcoholic kind without suffering for it the next day. So know some hangover cures and drink plenty of water before you fall asleep.

I

is for the improper inebriation and illicit insatiability of every good hedonist.

J

is for Jacuzzi; always more enjoyable with a partner or a group and a glass of chilled champagne.

K

is for kissing of course, and all its myriad forms and delicious combinations.

L

is for leather and lace, and libidinous lap-dancing.

M

is for music. From operatic arias through to head-banging thrash metal, there's something for every taste. Make a wild compilation tape for a party or a sentimental one for your lover.

N

is for negligée at night-time; there's nothing like traditional black lace to spice things up.

O

is for opulence. Minimalism is out, decadence is in. Spoil yourself with opulent food and furnishings and have a decadent social life.

P

is for perfume. Scents can dramatically affect your mood so use them to enhance your sexual, romantic or hedonistic feelings.

Q

is for quality and quantity: make sure that whatever you do to make your life special, there is lots of it and it is only of the best quality.

R

is for romance, roses and room service . . .

S

is for satin and silk. Use satin sheets on the bed for a touch of luxury at night-time and wear silk as often as you can.

T

is for touching; feel the benefits of a massage – to your relationship as well as your body.

U

is for underwear. It doesn't matter if no one is going to see it; wearing a tiger print thong will make you feel naughty all day!

V

is for Valentine. Treat your loved one as if every day was Valentine's Day.

W

is for water. Hot tubs, seasides, candle-lit baths – all are essential for the romantic in you.

X

is for X-rated. Indulge in erotic literature and sexy films to get inspiration for your own bedroom antics.

Y

is for yes, yes, yes! A hedonist never says no to even the most outlandish of suggestions.

Z

is for zest – whatever you choose to do in life, do it with vigour and panache.

BIBLIOGRAPHY

Classic Love Poems (2001, Summersdale)

Bryant, Mark **Private Lives** (1996, Cassell)

Crystal, David (ed.) **The Cambridge Biographical Dictionary** (1998, CUP)

Graves, Robert **The Greek Myths** (1992, Penguin)

Kaplan, Justin (ed.) **Bartlett's Familiar Quotations** (1992, Little, Brown and Company)

Knowles, Elizabeth **The Oxford Book of Quotations** (1999, OUP)

Love, Brenda **Encyclopaedia of Unusual Sexual Practices** (1998, Abacus)

Maxwell-Hudson, Clare **Aromatherapy Massage** (1994, Dorling Kindersley)

Tannahill, Reay **Sex in History** (1980, Stein and Day)

www.summersdale.com